Mi Diario

de Embarazo

A Keepsake Pregnancy Journal

By The Unedited You

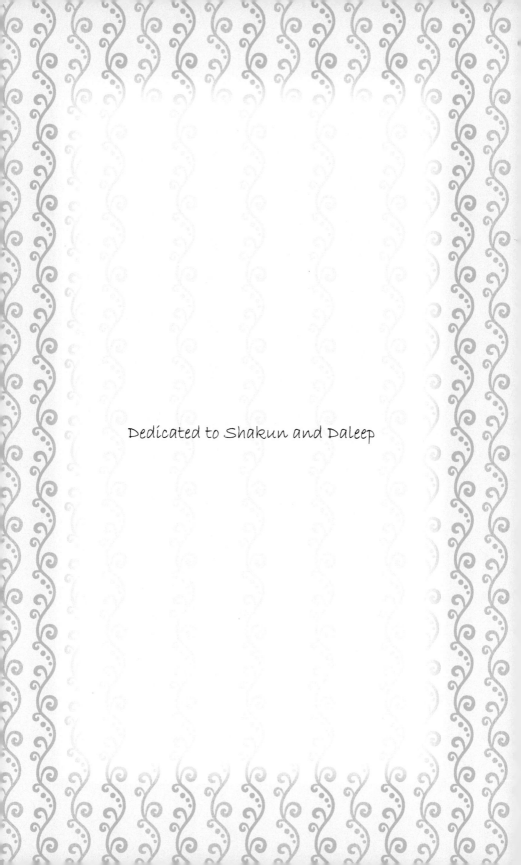

Dedicated to Shakun and Daleep

Acerca de mí

Mi nombre:_____

_____

Mi edad:_____

_____

Mi cumpleaños: _____

_____

Mi lugar de nacimiento: _____

_____

Mi signo zodiacal: _____

_____

El nombre de mi madre: _____

_____

El nombre de mi padre: _____

_____

El nombre de mi esposo:_____

_____

Mis hermanos:_____

_____

Mis pasatiempos _____

_____

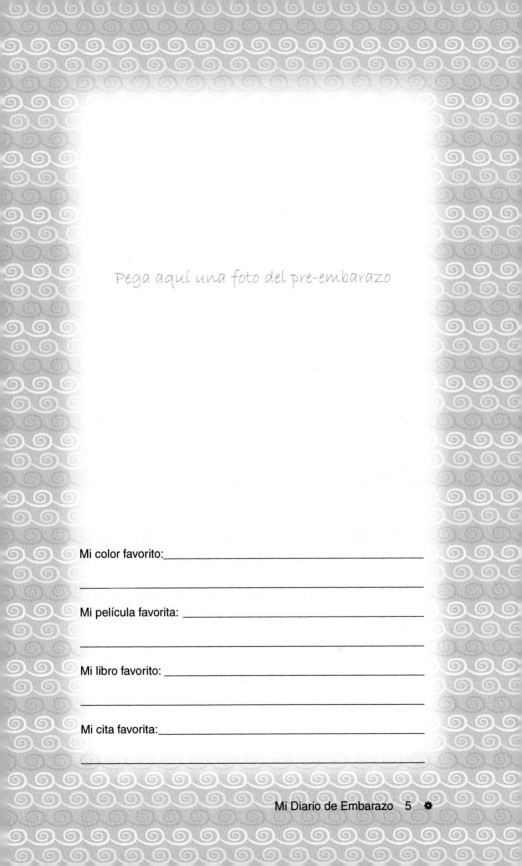

Pega aquí una foto del pre-embarazo

Mi color favorito:_____

_____

Mi película favorita: _____

_____

Mi libro favorito: _____

_____

Mi cita favorita:_____

_____

Pega aquí fotos de la familia

Las maravillosas noticias

Cuándo descubrí que estaba embarazada:_____

_____

Cómo lo descubrí: _____

_____

Dónde estaba: _____

_____

Mi reacción: _____

_____

Reacciones de mi familia: _____

_____

Fecha esperada de nacimiento: _____

_____

La mejor cualidad de mi madre: _____

_____

La mejor cualidad de mi padre: _____

_____

La mejor cualidad de mi esposo:_____

_____

Cualidades que quiero tenga mi bebé: _____

_____

Las primeras fotos del bebé: fotos del ultrasonido

Fecha y hora:_____

Semana de embarazo: _____

_____

_____

Mis pensamientos y sentimientos:_____

_____

_____

_____

_____

Pega aquí una foto del ultrasonido del bebé

Las primeras fotos del bebé: fotos del ultrasonido

Fecha y hora:_____

Semana de embarazo: _____

_____

_____

Mis pensamientos y sentimientos:_____

_____

_____

_____

_____

Pega aquí una foto del ultrasonido del bebé

¡Página de mis primeras veces!

Primera vez que escuché el latido del bebé:_____

Fecha y hora:_____

Mis emociones: _____

_____

_____

_____

_____

Primera vez que usé ropa de maternidad:_____

Fecha y hora:_____

Mis emociones: _____

_____

_____

_____

Primera vez que sentí una agitación o movimiento del bebé: _____

Fecha y hora:_____

Mis emociones: _____

_____

_____

_____

_____

¡Página de mis primeras veces!

Primera vez que sentí una patadita: _____

Fecha y hora: _____

Mis emociones: _____

_____

_____

_____

_____

_____

Primera vez que sentí una contracción: _____

Fecha y hora: _____

Mis emociones: _____

_____

_____

_____

Primera vez que vi/sostuve a mi bebé: _____

Fecha y hora: _____

Mis emociones: _____

_____

_____

_____

_____

¡Nombres que me gustan!

Nombres de niño

_____   _____
_____   _____
_____   _____
_____   _____
_____   _____
_____   _____
_____   _____

Nombres de niña

_____   _____
_____   _____
_____   _____
_____   _____
_____   _____
_____   _____
_____   _____

Primer Trimestre

Estás embarazada y eres poderosa.
Eres valiente y eres hermosa. Sigue
adelante con tu valentía, tu belleza
y tu conectividad. Confía en tu
cuerpo para dar a luz y saber que
el poder colectivo de las mujeres
del mundo estará contigo.
~Autor Desconocido

Semana 6

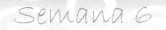

Pega aquí una foto de tu pancita de embarazo

Fecha: _____ Peso: _____

Medida del vientre: _____

Mis sentimientos/niveles de energía/disposición en general: _____

_____

_____

_____

_____

Un mensaje desde el corazón para mi bebé aún no nacido (esperanzas, sueños y aspiraciones): _____

_____

_____

_____

_____

Semana 7

Fecha: _____

Mis pensamientos: _____

_____

_____

_____

_____

Mis antojos y apetito: _____

_____

Aversiones: _____

_____

_____

La parte más memorable de la semana: _____

_____

_____

Otras notas: _____

_____

_____

_____

_____

_____

Semana 8

Fecha: _____

Mis pensamientos: _____

_____

_____

_____

_____

Mis antojos y apetito: _____

_____

Aversiones: _____

_____

_____

La parte más memorable de la semana: _____

_____

_____

Otras notas: _____

_____

_____

_____

_____

_____

Semana 9

Fecha: _____

Mis pensamientos:_____

_____

_____

_____

_____

Mis antojos y apetito:_____

_____

Aversiones: _____

_____

_____

La parte más memorable de la semana:_____

_____

_____

Otras notas:_____

_____

_____

_____

_____

_____

Semana 10

Fecha: _____

Mis pensamientos: _____

_____

_____

_____

_____

Mis antojos y apetito: _____

_____

Aversiones: _____

_____

_____

La parte más memorable de la semana: _____

_____

_____

Otras notas: _____

_____

_____

_____

_____

_____

Semana 11

Fecha: _____

Mis pensamientos: _____

_____

_____

_____

_____

Mis antojos y apetito: _____

_____

Aversiones: _____

_____

_____

La parte más memorable de la semana: _____

_____

_____

Otras notas: _____

_____

_____

_____

_____

_____

Semana 12

Fecha: _____

Mis pensamientos:_____

_____

_____

_____

_____

Mis antojos y apetito:_____

_____

Aversiones: _____

_____

_____

La parte más memorable de la semana:_____

_____

_____

Otras notas: _____

_____

_____

_____

_____

_____

SEGUNDO TRIMESTRE

La vida es una flama que siempre
se consume a sí misma, pero se
enciende cada vez que nace un bebé.
– George Bernard Shaw

Semana 13

Pega aquí una foto de tu pancita de embarazo

Fecha: _____Peso: _____

Medida del vientre: _____

Mis sentimientos/niveles de energía/disposición en general: _____

_____

_____

_____

_____

Un mensaje desde el corazón para mi bebé aún no nacido (esperanzas, sueños y aspiraciones): _____

_____

_____

_____

_____

Semana 14

Fecha: _____

Mis pensamientos:_____

_____

_____

_____

_____

La parte más memorable de la semana:_____

_____

_____

Otras notas:_____

_____

_____

_____

_____

_____

_____

_____

_____

_____

_____

Semana 15

Fecha: _____

Mis pensamientos: _____

_____

_____

_____

_____

La parte más memorable de la semana: _____

_____

_____

Otras notas: _____

_____

_____

_____

_____

_____

_____

_____

_____

Semana 16

Fecha: _____

Mis pensamientos:_____

_____

_____

_____

_____

La parte más memorable de la semana:_____

_____

_____

Otras notas: _____

_____

_____

_____

_____

_____

_____

_____

_____

_____

Semana 17

Pega aquí una foto de tu pancita de embarazo

Fecha: _____ Peso: _____

Medida del vientre: _____

Mis sentimientos/niveles de energía/disposición en general: _____

_____

_____

_____

_____

Un mensaje desde el corazón para mi bebé aún no nacido (esperanzas, sueños y aspiraciones): _____

_____

_____

_____

_____

Semana 18

Fecha: _____

Mis pensamientos: _____

_____

_____

_____

_____

La parte más memorable de la semana: _____

_____

_____

Otras notas: _____

_____

_____

_____

_____

_____

_____

_____

_____

_____

_____

_____

Semana 19

Fecha: _____

Mis pensamientos:_____

_____

_____

_____

_____

La parte más memorable de la semana:_____

_____

_____

Otras notas: _____

_____

_____

_____

_____

_____

_____

_____

_____

_____

_____

Semana 20

Fecha: _____

Mis pensamientos: _____

_____

_____

_____

_____

La parte más memorable de la semana: _____

_____

_____

Otras notas: _____

_____

_____

_____

_____

_____

_____

_____

_____

_____

_____

Semana 21

Pega aquí una foto de tu pancita de embarazo

Fecha: _____ Peso: _____

Medida del vientre: _____

Mis sentimientos/niveles de energía/disposición en general: _____

_____

_____

_____

_____

Un mensaje desde el corazón para mi bebé aún no nacido (esperanzas, sueños y aspiraciones): _____

_____

_____

_____

_____

Semana 22

Fecha: _____

Mis pensamientos:_____

_____

_____

_____

_____

La parte más memorable de la semana:_____

_____

_____

Otras notas:_____

_____

_____

_____

_____

_____

_____

_____

_____

_____

_____

_____

Semana 23

Fecha: _____

Mis pensamientos:_____

_____

_____

_____

_____

La parte más memorable de la semana: _____

_____

_____

Otras notas: _____

_____

_____

_____

_____

_____

_____

_____

_____

_____

_____

Semana 24

Fecha: _____

Mis pensamientos: _____

_____

_____

_____

_____

La parte más memorable de la semana: _____

_____

_____

Otras notas: _____

_____

_____

_____

_____

_____

_____

_____

_____

_____

_____

Semana 25

Pega aquí una foto de tu pancita de embarazo

Fecha: _____ Peso: _____

Medida del vientre: _____

Mis sentimientos/niveles de energía/disposición en general: _____

_____

_____

_____

_____

Un mensaje desde el corazón para mi bebé aún no nacido (esperanzas, sueños y aspiraciones): _____

_____

_____

_____

_____

Semana 26

Fecha: _____

Mis pensamientos: _____

_____

_____

_____

_____

La parte más memorable de la semana: _____

_____

_____

Otras notas: _____

_____

_____

_____

_____

_____

_____

_____

_____

_____

_____

Semana 27

Fecha: _____

Mis pensamientos:_____

_____

_____

_____

_____

La parte más memorable de la semana:_____

_____

_____

Otras notas:_____

_____

_____

_____

_____

_____

_____

_____

_____

_____

_____

_____

_____

Semana 28

Fecha: _____

Mis pensamientos:_____

_____

_____

_____

_____

La parte más memorable de la semana: _____

_____

_____

Otras notas:_____

_____

_____

_____

_____

_____

_____

_____

_____

_____

_____

Tercer Trimestre

El embarazo toma los miedos
más profundos de una mujer
y le demuestra que es más
fuerte de lo que ella pensaba.
~ Anónimo

¡Mi Baby Shower!

Pega aquí fotos del baby shower

Fecha: _____

Notas: _____

_____

_____

_____

Lista de cosas para la maleta del hospital

PARA EL BEBÉ

☐ Pañales de recién nacido

☐ Toallitas húmedas

☐ Trajecitos de una pieza para recién nacidos

☐ Chalecos de recién nacido

☐ Gorros y calcetines

☐ Cojín de lactancia

☐ Cobija de recepción

PARA MAMITA

☐ Cepillo y pasta de dientes

☐ Limpiador de rostro

☐ Crema humectante

☐ Maquillaje (¡para las fotos!)

☐ Toalla pequeña

☐ Brasier de lactancia y almohadillas para pechos

☐ Bata o ropa cómoda y calcetines

☐ Suéter o Jersey

☐ Cargador de teléfono

☐ Copia del registro médico y prenatal

Semana 29

Pega aquí una foto de tu pancita de embarazo

Fecha: _____Peso: _____

Medida del vientre: _____

Mis sentimientos/niveles de energía/disposición en general: _____

_____

_____

_____

_____

Un mensaje desde el corazón para mi bebé aún no nacido (esperanzas, sueños y aspiraciones): _____

_____

_____

_____

_____

Semana 30

Fecha: _____

¿Cómo me siento?? _____

_____

_____

_____

_____

_____

Otros comentarios: _____

_____

_____

_____

_____

_____

_____

_____

_____

_____

_____

Semana 31

Fecha: _____

¿Cómo me siento?? _____

_____

_____

_____

_____

_____

Otros comentarios: _____

_____

_____

_____

_____

_____

_____

_____

_____

_____

_____

_____

_____

Semana 32

DFecha: _____

¿Cómo me siento?? _____

_____

_____

_____

_____

_____

Otros comentarios: _____

_____

_____

_____

_____

_____

_____

_____

_____

_____

_____

Semana 33

Pega aquí una foto de tu pancita de embarazo

Fecha: _____Peso: _____

Medida del vientre: _____

Mis sentimientos/niveles de energía/disposición en general: _____

_____

_____

_____

_____

Un mensaje desde el corazón para mi bebé aún no nacido (esperanzas, sueños y aspiraciones): _____

_____

_____

_____

_____

Semana 34

Fecha: _____

¿Cómo me siento?? _____

_____

_____

_____

_____

_____

Otros comentarios: _____

_____

_____

_____

_____

_____

_____

_____

_____

_____

_____

_____

_____

Semana 35

Fecha: _____

¿Cómo me siento?? _____

_____

_____

_____

_____

_____

Otros comentarios: _____

_____

_____

_____

_____

_____

_____

_____

_____

_____

_____

_____

Semana 36

Fecha: _____

¿Cómo me siento?? _____

_____

_____

_____

_____

_____

Otros comentarios: _____

_____

_____

_____

_____

_____

_____

_____

_____

_____

_____

_____

Semana 37

Pega aquí una foto de tu pancita de embarazo

Fecha: _____ Peso: _____

Medida del vientre: _____

Mis sentimientos/niveles de energía/disposición en general: _____

_____

_____

_____

_____

Un mensaje desde el corazón para mi bebé aún no nacido (esperanzas, sueños y aspiraciones): _____

_____

_____

_____

_____

Semana 38

Fecha: _____

¿Cómo me siento?? _____

_____

_____

_____

_____

_____

Otros comentarios: _____

_____

_____

_____

_____

_____

_____

_____

_____

_____

_____

_____

Semana 39

Fecha: _____

¿Cómo me siento?? _____

_____

_____

_____

_____

_____

Otros comentarios: _____

_____

_____

_____

_____

_____

_____

_____

_____

_____

_____

_____

_____

_____

_____

Semana 40

Pega aquí una foto de tu pancita de embarazo

Fecha: _____ Peso: _____

Medida del vientre: _____

Mis sentimientos/niveles de energía/disposición en general: _____

_____

_____

_____

_____

Un mensaje desde el corazón para mi bebé aún no nacido (esperanzas, sueños y aspiraciones): _____

_____

_____

_____

_____

Parto y nacimiento

Pega aquí una foto de tu recién nacido

Fecha y hora que entré en labor:_____

Cuánto duró mi parto: _____

Reflecciones: _____

_____

Fecha y hora de la llegada del bebé:_____

Niño o niña: _____

Peso: _____

Altura: _____

Tipo de sangre: _____

Quién recibió al bebé: _____

Quién estaba presente a la hora del nacimiento del bebé: _____

_____

_____

Mirando hacia pasado: reflexiones acerca de mi pancita de embarazada

_____

_____

_____

_____

_____

_____

_____

_____

_____

_____

_____

_____

_____

_____

_____